Liquid THC

How to Make Easy Delicious Marijuana Infused Drinks for
Medical Marijuana Users

Cara knights

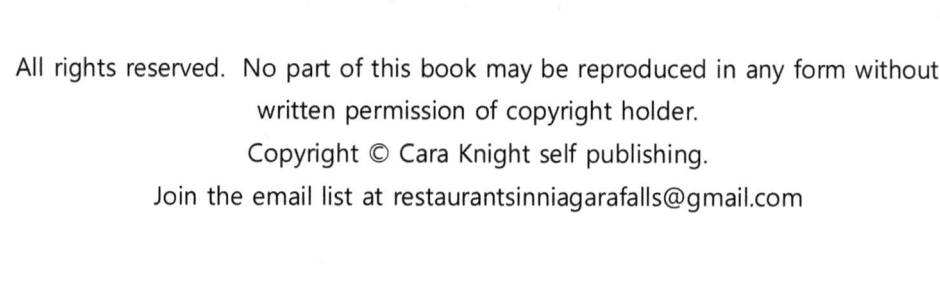

Table of contents

NOTE: This book is intended for medical marijuana users to give alternatives on consuming the product. Please enjoy responsibly.

Book Background

Welcome to Liquid THC. Inside you'll find great drink ideas using marijuana.

I started cooking with cannabis when my husband developed chronic insomnia after having started dialysis. (Apparently one of the side affects.) After about 3 years of over the counter medication and various prescriptions that left him feeling worse in the morning I knew I had to find something that worked. After doing some research I discovered that marijuana also can be used as a sleep aid. And the testimonials I read were inspiring.

We immediately contacted my husband's dialysis Dr. who then recommended a Cannabis Dr for us to see.

Seeing as how my husband does not smoke and didn't want to start now I had to find another way for him to take the cannabis, and I did!

My husband now enjoys a small cup of cannabis tea every night at least two hours before bed. After a year of cannabis tea, he now has a long restful sleep and wakes up refreshed and ready to start the day. This is what has inspired me to put this book together and share with you.

So please cook and enjoy!

Drinks

Main Cannabis Solution

Ingredients:
- ❖ Large mason jar filled with chopped cannabis leaves, stems and buds
- ❖ Bottle of (your choice) tequila, vodka or rum

Directions:
- ❖ Add tequila to chopped cannabis jar. Shake and let sit for 1-2 weeks. (shake occasionally)
- ❖ After desired sit time, strain into another bottle to keep until needed.

Note: Refrigerate

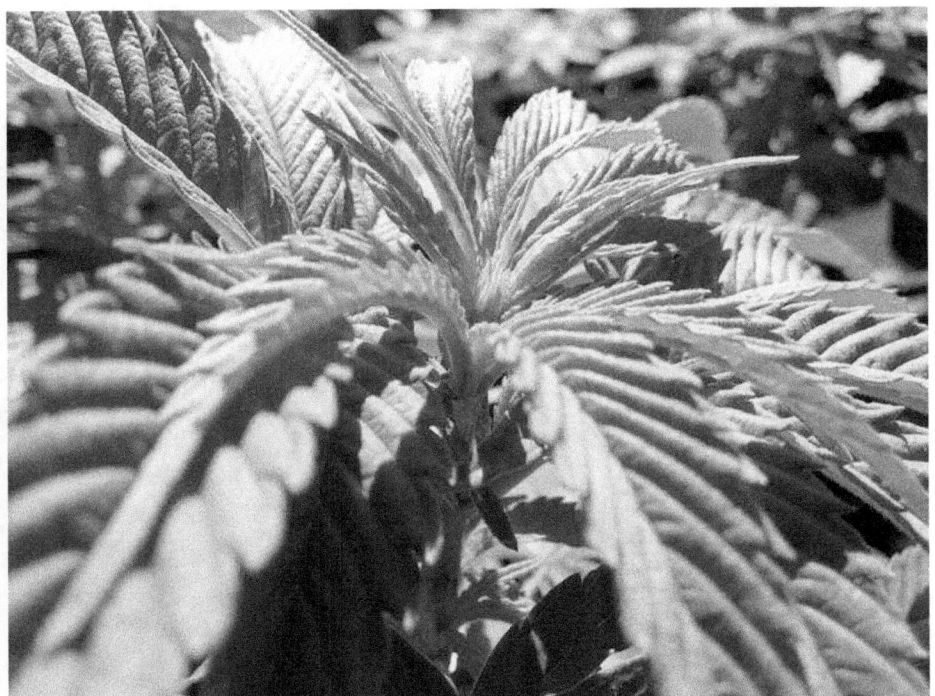

Blitzed Breezer

Ingredients
- ❖ 1.5oz Main Cannabis Solution (see recipe)
- ❖ Old Fashion Glass
- ❖ Grapefruit Juice
- ❖ 1oz. Cranberry Juice

Directions
- ❖ Fill glass with ice
- ❖ Add 1.5 oz cannabis solution
- ❖ Fill glass with grapefruit juice
- ❖ Add cranberry juice

Note: Gently stir and enjoy

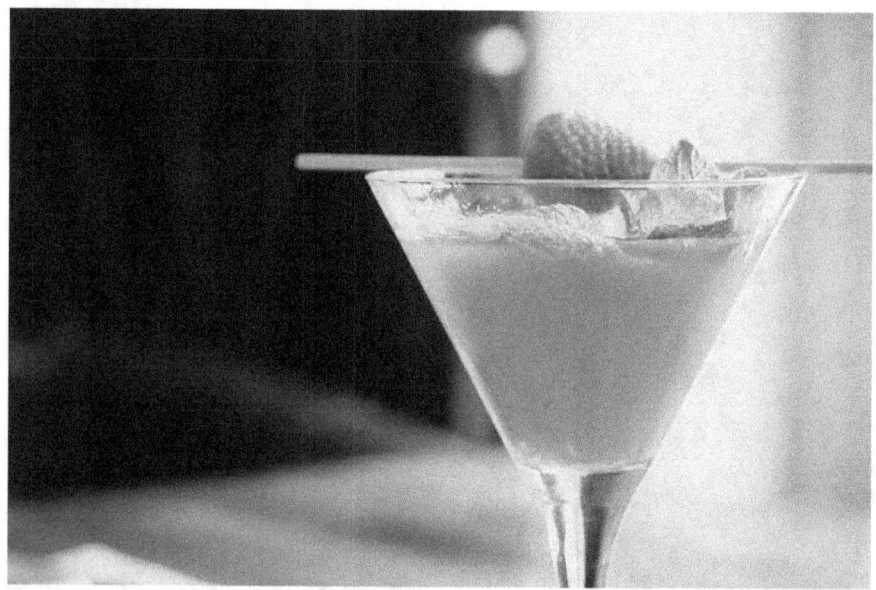

The Blue Zone

Ingredients
- ❖ 1 oz. Main Cannabis Solution (see recipe)
- ❖ 2 oz. Pineapple Juice
- ❖ 1 oz. Blue Curacao
- ❖ 1 oz. Coconut Crème
- ❖ 1 Slice Pineapple
- ❖ 1 Cherry
- ❖ High Ball Glass

Directions
- ❖ Blend together main cannabis solution, blue curacao, pineapple juice, and coconut crème with one cup ice in an electric mixer at high speed
- ❖ Pour into a highball glass.
- ❖ Decorate with the slice of pineapple and a cherry.

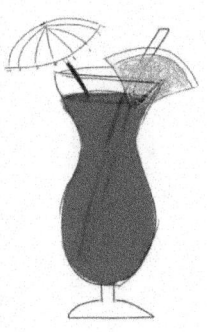

Loaded with Fruit

Ingredients
- ❖ 2 oz. Main Cannabis Solution (see recipe)
- ❖ 1 oz. White Rum
- ❖ 2 oz. Lime Juice
- ❖ 3 oz. Passion Fruit Juice
- ❖ 2 oz. Pineapple Juice
- ❖ 1 oz. Orange Juice
- ❖ 1 Tbsp. Grenadine
- ❖ Highball Glass

Directions
- ❖ Fill a cocktail shaker with ice
- ❖ Add all the ingredients
- ❖ Cover, and shake well, Strain into a highball glass
- ❖ Garnish with a slice of pineapple and cherry

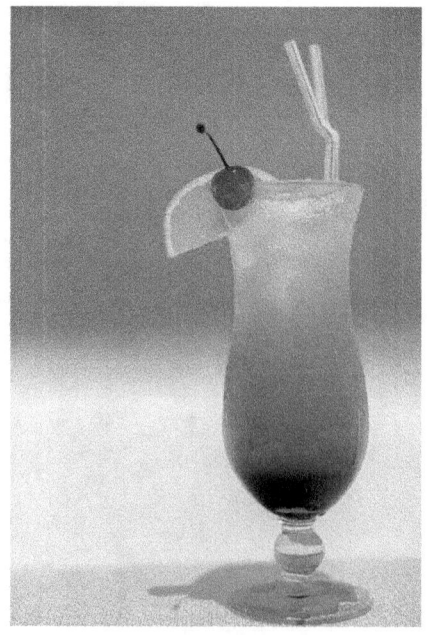

Red Eye Cranberry Cocktail

Ingredients
- ❖ ½ Cup Cold Water
- ❖ 2 oz. Cranberry Juice Chilled
- ❖ 3 oz. Lemonade Juice
- ❖ 4 oz. Main Cannabis Solution (see recipe)
- ❖ Cocktail Glass

Directions
- ❖ Combine the first 3 ingredients in a mixer
- ❖ Mix well
- ❖ Add cannabis solution, stir gently.
- ❖ Enjoy

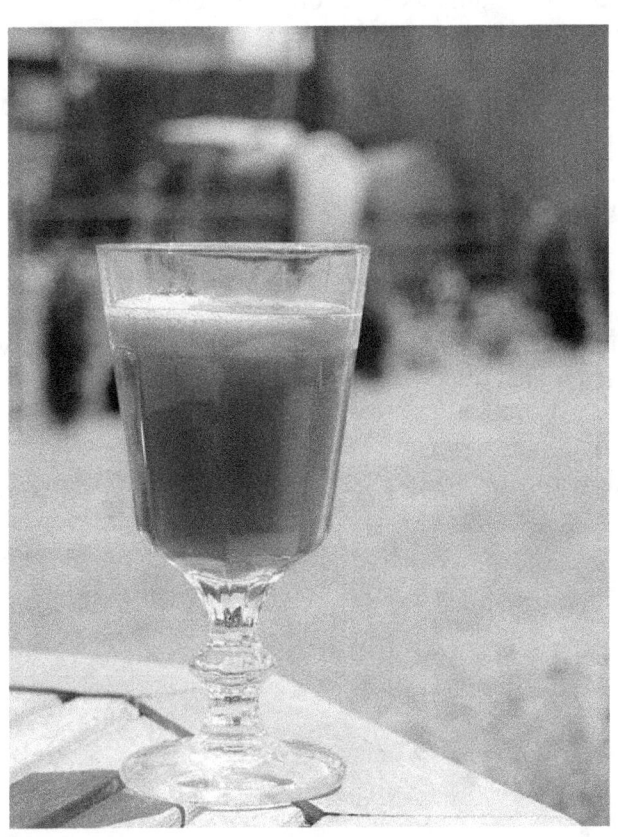

SMOOTHIES

Happy High Strawberry Smoothie

Ingredients

- ❖ 1 Cup Main Cannabis Solution (see recipe)
- ❖ 1/2 tsp. Lime Juice
- ❖ 1 tsp. Orange Juice
- ❖ 3 Fresh Strawberries
- ❖ 2 Scoops Strawberry Sorbet
- ❖ Crushed ice
- ❖ Margarita Glass

Directions

- ❖ Place the cannabis solution, lime juice, orange juice, strawberries and strawberry sorbet into your smoothie blender
- ❖ Process until smooth.
- ❖ Pour over ice and serve.
- ❖ Decorate with strawberry slices.

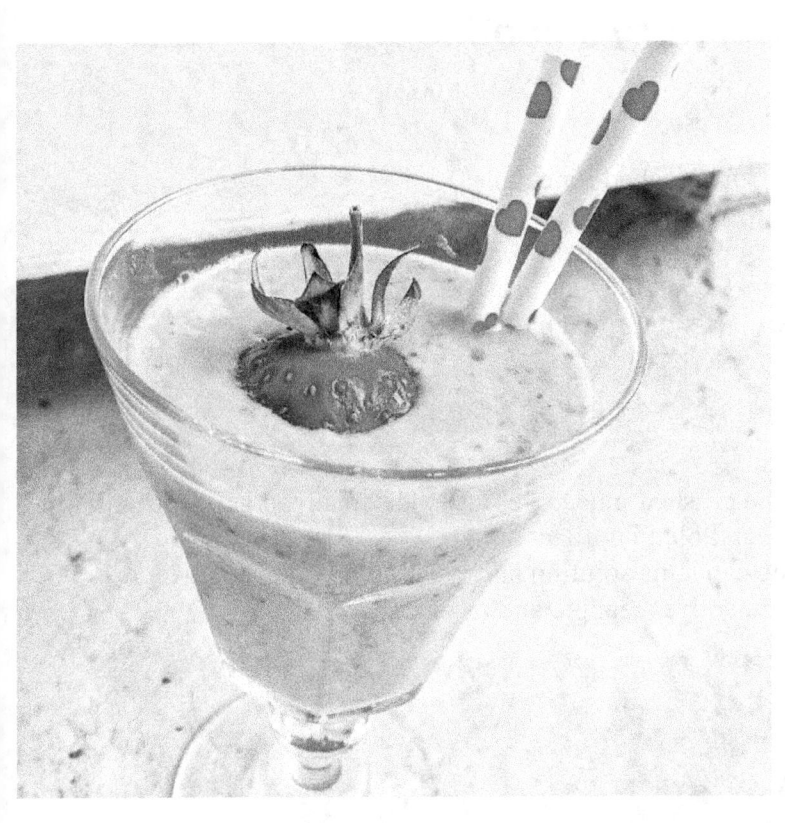

Smookin' Creamy Smoothie

Ingredients

- ❖ 3/4 Cup Crushed Pineapple
- ❖ 1 Cup Whole Milk
- ❖ 2 Scoops Vanilla Ice Cream
- ❖ 2 tbsp Coconut Milk
- ❖ ½ Cup Main Cannabis Solution (see recipe)
- ❖ Cherry to Decorate

Directions

- ❖ Place the crushed pineapple, milk, ice cream and coconut milk into blender and blend until smooth.
- ❖ Add the cannabis solution and blend to mix thoroughly.
- ❖ Decorate with pineapple and or cherry.

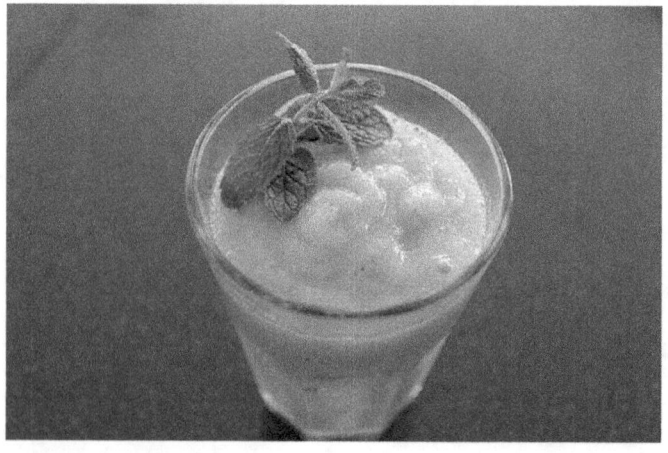

Zoned Out Pineapple Mango Smoothie

Ingredients
- ❖ 1 Cup mango, diced (can use frozen)
- ❖ 1 Cup Frozen Pineapple
- ❖ 3 Limes Juiced
- ❖ 2/3 Cups Cannabis Solution (see recipe)
- ❖ ¼ Cup Triple Sec

Directions
- ❖ Place the mango, pineapple, lime juice, cannabis solution and triple sec into a blender. Blend until smooth.
- ❖ Serve immediately in salt rimmed glasses.

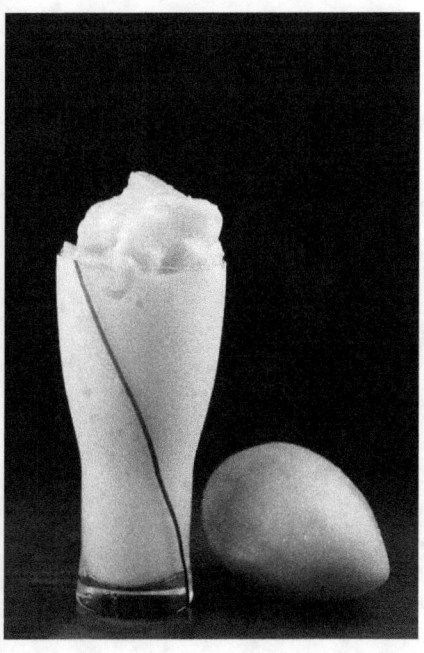

Loaded Orange Smoothie

Ingredients

- ❖ 1/2 orange (peeled)
- ❖ Crushed ice
- ❖ 1/2 Cup Main Cannabis Solution (see recipe)

Directions

- ❖ Put the orange and ice in the blender and blend until smooth.
- ❖ Add main cannabis solution and blend
- ❖ Pour over crushed ice

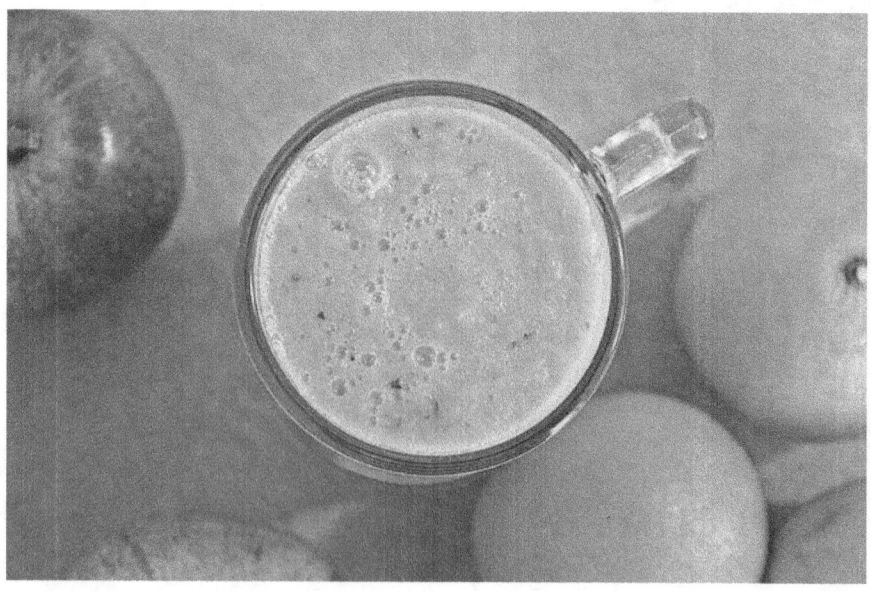

Blitzed Out Peach Smoothie

Ingredients

- ❖ ½ Cup main cannabis solution (see recipe)
- ❖ 1/2 Cup orange juice
- ❖ 1 Tablespoon cream of coconut
- ❖ 2 Cups frozen peaches
- ❖ 1 Tablespoon sugar
- ❖ 2 Cups ice cubes

Directions

- ❖ Add all of the ingredients to blender and blend until smooth.

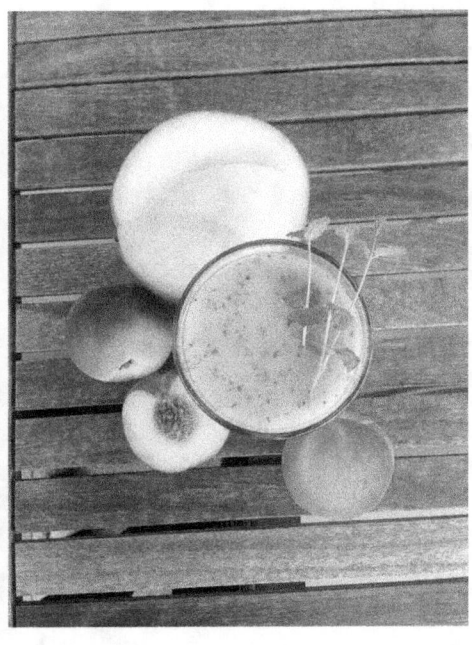

Blueberry Fields Smoothie

Ingredients
- ❖ ½ cup main cannabis solution
- ❖ 2 teaspoons cocoa powder
- ❖ 1 cup milk
- ❖ 4 tablespoons frozen blueberries
- ❖ 1 teaspoon white sugar
- ❖ 4 ice cubes

Directions

Mix together the cocoa powder and water in a small bowl until cocoa is dissolved.

Place the main cannabis solution, cocoa mixture, milk, blueberries, sugar and ice cubes into a blender, blend until smooth.

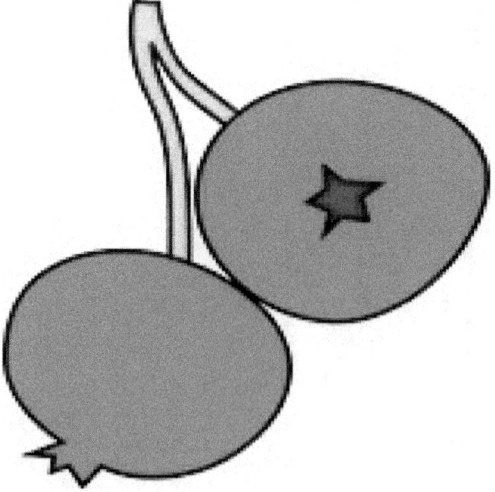

Peaches and Dreams Smoothie

Ingredients

- ❖ ½ cup main cannabis solution
- ❖ 1 can sliced peaches
- ❖ 4 scoops vanilla ice cream
- ❖ 2 cups vanilla soy milk
- ❖ ¼ cup orange juice

Directions
Blend together all above ingredients until smooth. Pour into glass and enjoy

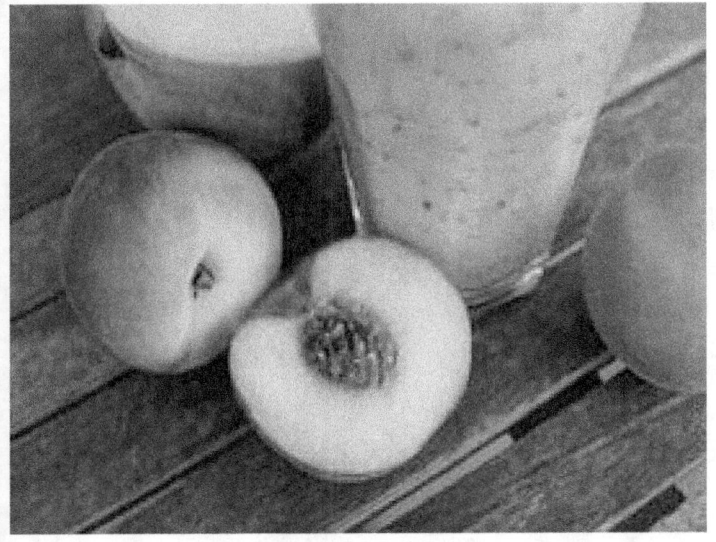

California Dreaming Smoothie

Ingredients

- ❖ ½ cup main cannabis solution
- ❖ 7 large strawberries
- ❖ 1 container lemon yogurt
- ❖ 1/3 cup orange juice

Directions

Place strawberries in a plastic container and freeze for an hour.

In a blender, combine frozen strawberries, yogurt and orange juice. Blend until smooth. Pour and serve.

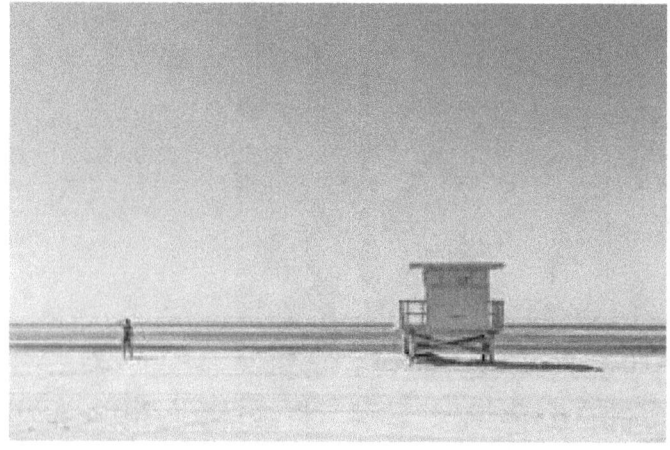

Fruity Red Eyes Smoothie

Ingredients

- ❖ ½ cup main cannabis solution
- ❖ 1 container strawberry yogurt
- ❖ ½ cup cranberry juice
- ❖ 1 ½ cups frozen strawberries, quartered
- ❖ 1 cup frozen raspberries
- ❖ 1 teaspoon sugar

Direction
Blend together yogurt, cranberry juice. Add strawberries, raspberries and sugar. Blend until smooth. Pour into glass and enjoy.

High Life Orange Smoothie

Ingredients

- ❖ 1 can frozen orange juice concentrate
- ❖ 1 cup milk
- ❖ ½ cup main cannabis solution
- ❖ 1 teaspoon vanilla extract
- ❖ 1/3 cup white sugar
- ❖ 10 ice cubes

Directions

In a blender, combine orange juice concentrate, milk, water, vanilla sugar and ice. Blend until smooth. Pour and enjoy.

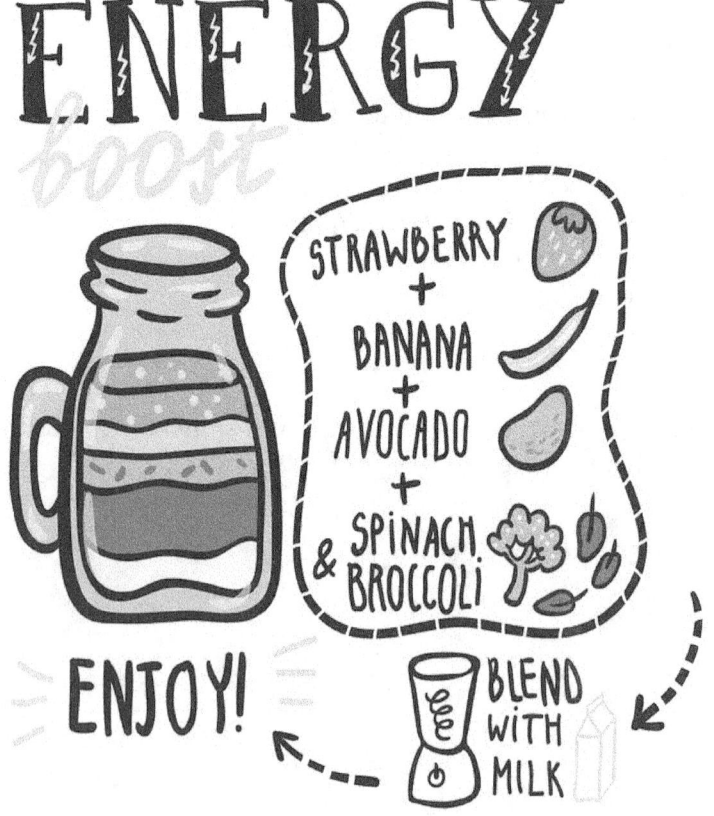

Note: Add ½ cup main cannabis solution

Kiwi Strawberry Happy Smoothie

Ingredients

- ½ cup main cannabis solution
- 1 banana
- 6 strawberries
- 1 kiwi
- ½ cup vanilla frozen yogurt
- ¾ cup pineapple and orange juice blend

Directions

Place banana, strawberries, kiwi, vanilla frozen yogurt and pineapple and orange juice blend in a blender. Blend until smooth.

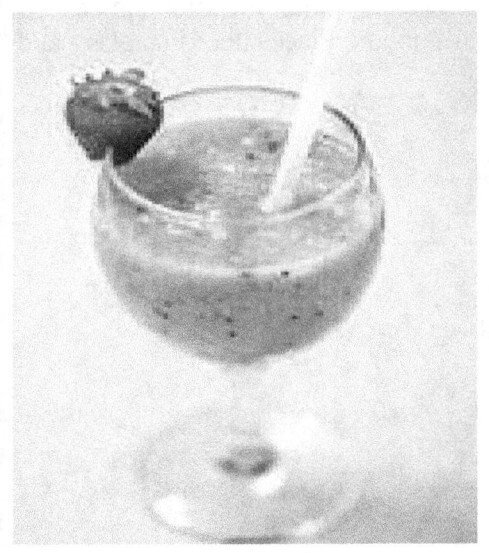

Honey-Mango Everything Funny Smoothie

Ingredients

- ❖ 1 mango peeled and cubed
- ❖ 1 tablespoon white sugar
- ❖ 2 tablespoons honey
- ❖ 1 cup nonfat milk
- ❖ 1 teaspoon lemon juice
- ❖ 1 cup ice cubes
- ❖ ½ cup main cannabis solution

Directions

Place the mango, sugar and honey in a blender, pour in the milk, lemon juice, and cannabis solution, blend until smooth. Place cubes in a glass, and pour mango smoothie over ice. Enjoy.

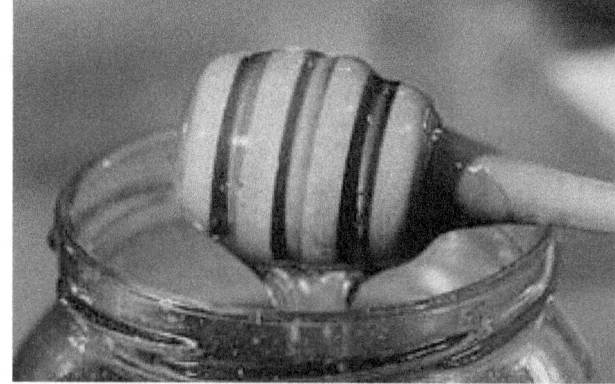

Chill Out Lemon Berry Smoothie

Ingredients

- ❖ 1 container blueberry nonfat yogurt
- ❖ 1 ½ cups skim milk
- ❖ 1 cup ice cubes
- ❖ 1 cup fresh blueberries
- ❖ 1 cup fresh strawberries
- ❖ 1 teaspoon powdered lemonade mix
- ❖ ½ cup main cannabis solution

Directions

Place yogurt, milk, ice cubes, blueberries, strawberries, and lemonade mix in a blender. Pulse until smooth and creamy.

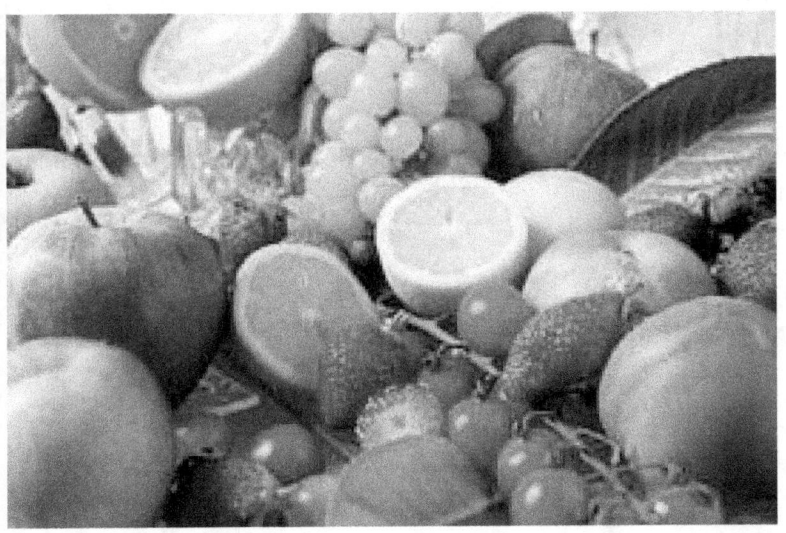

Groovy Smoothie

Ingredients

- ❖ 2 small bananas, broken into chunks
- ❖ 1 cup frozen strawberries
- ❖ 1 container vanilla low fat yogurt
- ❖ ¾ cup milk
- ❖ ½ cup main cannabis solution

Direction

In a blender, combine bananas, frozen strawberries, yogurt and milk. Blend until smooth. Enjoy.

Tropical Dream Smoothie

Ingredients

- ❖ 1 mango. Peeled and seeded
- ❖ 1 papaya, peeled and seeded
- ❖ ½ cup fresh strawberries
- ❖ 1/3 cup orange juice
- ❖ 5 ice cubes
- ❖ ½ cup main cannabis solution

Directions

Place the mango, papaya, strawberries, orange juice, and ice cubes in a blender. Process until the ingredients are smooth.

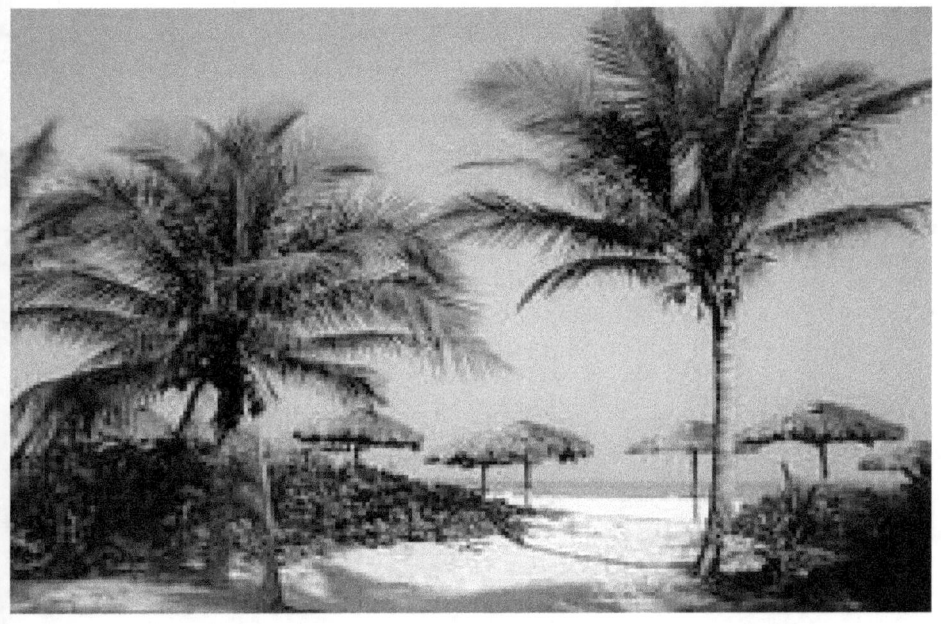

www.ingramcontent.com/pod-product-compliance
Lightning Source LLC
Chambersburg PA
CBHW070342190526
45169CB00005B/2011